Bulletproof Diet

*Lose Weight and Gain
Maximum Energy the
Bulletproof Way*

Table of Contents

Introduction

The book aims towards not only bringing to the fore the impending crisis regarding the diet of the average American but also towards providing adequate knowledge on the various types of food availability for the satisfaction of a healthy individual living in the 21st Century.

Through illustrative diagrams and by use of data available for the scrutiny of not only individuals but organizations as well and research substantiated by tangible evidence it became imperative that a book specifically designed for the analysis of such detrimental factors to the well-being of a nation.

Diet and nutrition is important for any individual seeking to fulfill his or her life goals and equally for any country aiming to achieve its targets. Proper nutrition can only be achieved through proper education- a goal made manifest and hopefully achieved through the strict compilation of the book the reader is about to enjoy.

Further, even though a good number of individuals composing the general human population knows a thing or two concerning the make-up of individual foods, the character and the professional acuity to compile their knowledge into a practicable entity becomes difficult hence necessitating the professional guidance of statistical emphasis.

Although it is important to start with the already disfigured population of adults in the current state of the nation, it is also necessary to deal with the younger population majorly because values and habits are instilled not from a developed stage, but from a developing stage. As most diseases related to the application of improper diets seem to affect the adult, it is evident now that these detriments tend to make themselves evident right from the time one is still young. Cases of increased cardiovascular ailments can therefore be put in check by the efforts of both individuals and parents guiding the eating habits of their young one from falling into the same pit they now find themselves in.

The Bulletproof Diet aims in as little space as possible highlight the gravity of the situation the country finds itself in at the present moment. Anyone reading through the book will definitely find the need to alter his or her dietary timetables and in turn take a keen look at the way he or she is exposing himself or herself to the dangers of a fragile body and system.

Chapter 1: Introduction into the Book

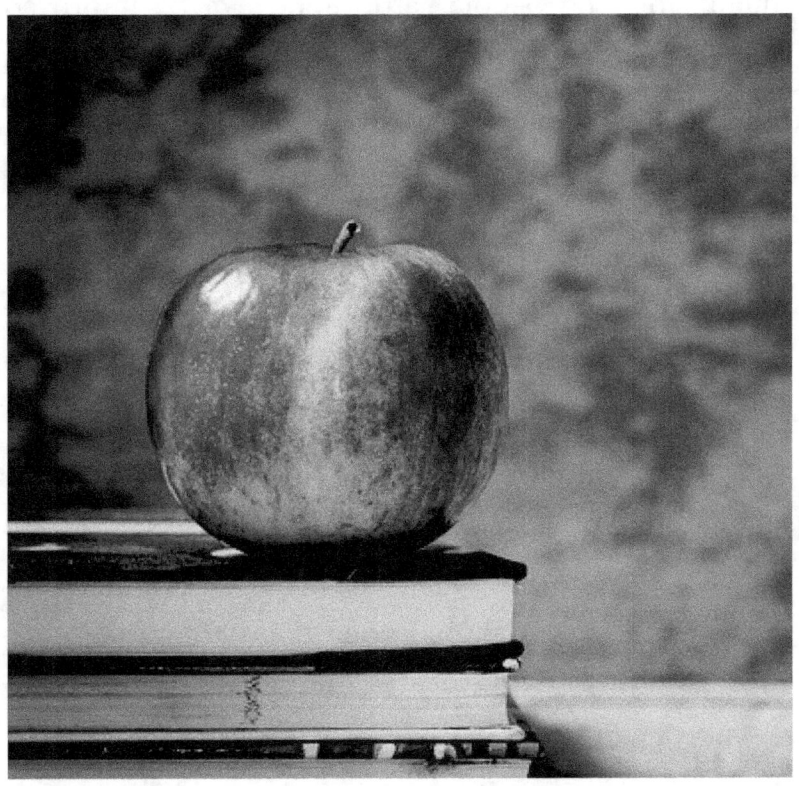

Out of ignorance or perhaps a mere lack of interest, most meals people enjoy is simply a smorgasbord of food that is quite low in the nutrients expected. Such foods are more quantity than quality. Even though most people can afford a healthy diet, they choose not to have one. It is necessary therefore that people are educated on what they should eat and what they should avoid. It is only through this means that the quality of food people settle upon can be improved and such level of education can only be spread using all available media including this one.

The benefits healthy food acquires a human being cannot be underestimated. One needs healthy foods for strong bones, higher levels of immunity and also for the health and well-being of one's brain. Without proper nutrition, the brain can be starved; hence, it is necessary to know not just what food to eat at any given time, but for what purpose one is consuming the food he or she is. This book should be able to make that manifest and should open the learner's mind to new territories with regard to food and the variety of options one has with regard to it.

The content in the book may as well come off as recommendations for a healthy diet. There are two overarching concepts; however, that need to be understood:

1) To achieve and sustain a healthy balance, one needs to maintain a balance of the calorie intake over time

Healthy people maintain their body weight and their shape through the intake of only balanced calories and ensure enough physical exercise burns up the extra calories. To help most people facing the obesity problem, most people must sacrifice themselves into trying to reduce the calorie they intake and expend event more of it in whatever way possible or is available.

2) People should focus on maintaining a nutrient dense food. Currently, there is too much sodium and too many calories in the average American diet coming from solid fats, added sugars and refined grain. These types of foods have come to be common place in the food outlets in America and have slowly replaced conventional nutritious food as was known before.

These two points could as well summarize the need and the purpose of this book. This book aims to provide information with regard to the best and the most nutritious meal alternatives. It aims to deepen the reader's knowledge with regard to what he or she should have at his dinner table or better yet, his breakfast table. In doing so, it helps craft a timetable not only for the use of the reader but also create a meal pattern for the same.

It is not enough for a healthy food pattern to create a healthy body but it should also focus on reducing the risk of contracting chronic diseases. Such diseases may arise out of improper cleaning procedures and careless disregard of standards of hygiene. In this regard, food should be first cleaned, separated, cooked and then chilled. This makes it proper for eating. Some foods may be detrimental to the individual when undercooked with these examples being milk, cheeses and juices that may have not been properly pasteurized. These pose risks to the individuals- risks of contracting what are commonly called foodborne diseases.

There comes to be key recommendations that come to arise with regard to this matter and these are as outlined below:

1) Balancing calories to manage weight.

- Improved eating and physical activities should help improve on overweight and obesity

- The total calorie intake should be controlled to manage the body weight of the person. For those who are overweight or obese, this would mean consuming lesser calories from the foods and beverages they intake.

- Increase engagement in physical activities and reduce the portion of time they spend daily on sedentary activities.

- During each stage of life, one should maintain a steady balance in calories throughout be it during childhood or during breastfeeding, during adolescence or during pregnancy.

2) Foods and components to reduce

- Reduce the intake of sodium to less than 2300 milligrams a day and further cut down the intake to less than 1500mg a day for those that are above the age of 51 or those belonging to any other age bracket but have hypertension, diabetes or chronic heart disease. Astonishingly, this applies to almost half of the population of the United States of America.

- Consume less than ten percent of calories from fatty acids that are saturated with monounsaturated and polyunsaturated fatty acids.

- Dietary cholesterol is to be consumed at a quantity of 300 mg a day

- Keep transfatty acid consumption as low as possible by reducing the intake of foods that contain synthetic sources of transfats which include partially hydrogenated oils.

- One is to reduce his or her intake of calories coming from solid fats and added sugars

- Limit the consumption of food that contains refined grains especially refined grain foods that contain solid fats and added sugars

- Alcohol should be consumed in moderation if it must be consumed and only by people of legal age

Foods and Nutrients to Increase

While restricting themselves within their calorie needs, individuals should maintain these recommendations while staying in the strict boundaries of a healthy eating pattern.

- Increase vegetable and fruit intake while staying within a healthy and diverse vegetable diet

- Replacing refined grains with whole grains – keeping this measurement in check by ensuring that one consumes as much as half of all the grains in his or her diet specifically being whole grains.

- One should increase the consumption of fat free or low fat milk and milk products including cheese, yoghurt and fortified soy beverages.

- Choose a variety of protein foods including sea food, lean meat, poultry, eggs, meat, soy products, unsalted nuts and seeds

- One should increase the amount of seafood consumed by choosing seafood in place of some meat and poultry

- Replace solid fats with oil where possible

- Foods that contain potassium, calcium, vitamin D and dietary fibre should be given priority since these are the most common elements missing in the average American diet.

Below are food choice recommendations suited to the group a particular individual belongs:

Women capable of becoming pregnant:

- For this group, it would be appropriate to have a rich supply of heme iron which is readily absorbed by the body of the women.

- This group also needs to consume a total of 400 micrograms a day of synthetic folic acid which can either come from fortified foods or supplements in addition to food forms of folate from a varied diet

Pregnant or Breastfeeding Women

- Consume foods fortified with vitamin B12, such as fortified cereals or dietary supplements

Building Healthy Eating Patterns

- Selecting an eating pattern that meets the nutrient needs of the person over time

- Account for all foods consumed and beverages and assess how they are to fit in the eating schedule

- Follow food safety recommendations while preparing food so as to reduce the risks of food related diseases

The ultimate aim of the book here is to provide a concise dietary plan for those who intend to keep an eye on their weight as well as their intake of nutrition. Poor diet and physical inactivity are the main causes of an obese generation. Without physical exercise, one can contract cardiovascular diseases, hypertension, hypertension, osteoporosis and other common diseases.

Recent surveys have come to suggest that as much as 15 percent of American households lack the sufficient income to acquire the right food and hence the right nutrition. Other parts of the population, even though they can afford a whole meal, go on to consume less of what they should consume were it to be compared to the recommended levels of intake.

Children are an important focus in the documentation of this type of diet because their stage in the development of the adult man is crucial in every way. In addition to that, most of the risk factors associated with chronic diseases are seen to have started becoming manifest in the younger ages. It is also common for people to carry forward their eating habits up to their older ages thereby making the early interruption of eating habits a huge priority.

The Heavy Toll of Diet Related Chronic Diseases (as of 2010)

Cardiovascular Disease- About 37% of the population has cardiovascular disease. The major risk factors of the diseases include tobacco use, hypertension, type 2 diabetes and obesity.

Hypertension- 34 % of US adults have hypertension. It is a major risk factor for heart disease, stroke, failure of the heart and kidney disease. About 16% of the American population is at risk of prehypertension.

Diabetes – In the United states, about 11% of the population suffers from diabetes whereas about 35% of the population is in the prediabetic stage. This is a stage where the blood sugar levels are a little higher than normal but at the same time not at that stage one can be called a diabetic.

However, it should be emphasized that the group which is affected most by the diabetics' statistics is that whose ages are above 20 years of old.

Cancer- Almost one in two men and women, it has been found, will be diagnosed with cancer ultimately. That interprets as up to 41 percent of the population.

Osteoporosis- One out of every two men and one in every four men will have contracted osteoporosis during their lifetime. This is statistic for those men above the ages of 50. About 80% of the bone mass in girls is acquired at the age of eighteen whereas in boys it is acquired at the age of 20.

The book is organized into the following sections:

Describes the factors relating to calorie balance and obesity. It also goes ahead to discuss diet and exercises related to the physique of the individual.

Foods and Food Components to Reduce: this section is dedicated to the food components that Americans take in large proportions in relation to the recommended amounts of the said food components.

Foods and Nutrients to Increase: In this section, there is covered the foods that one ought to increase in the diet one chooses. This includes those foods that are fat free and with low milk content and those high in potassium as well- as has been mentioned before.

Building Healthy Eating Pattern: This entails the combining of the nutrition recommendations into a steady pattern to be obeyed by the one willing to create better nutrition patterns.

Helping People make Healthy Choices: The ultimate goal of this book is to guide the American through the best nutrition pattern for one's employ. This helps make it easier even for the adoption of future generations into the ultimate nutritious diet. This step; however, has to be followed up into the remotest of regions the most common American may be living in.

The material and the content to be found in this book is to be and can be applied by various areas of government and the various departments dedicated to the welfare of the society. This includes the educational institutions, health institutions and even religious institutions considering that religions (most, if not all of them) exalt the purity of the body as much as that of the soul.

Our knowledge concerning nutrition continues to grow yet surprising our eating pattern does not seem to have any difference in the period that has elapsed. More than has ever been necessary, consumers in the present age need a sound and professional advice on the kind of meals to have and the content in that meal.

Chapter 2: Balancing Calories to Manage Weight

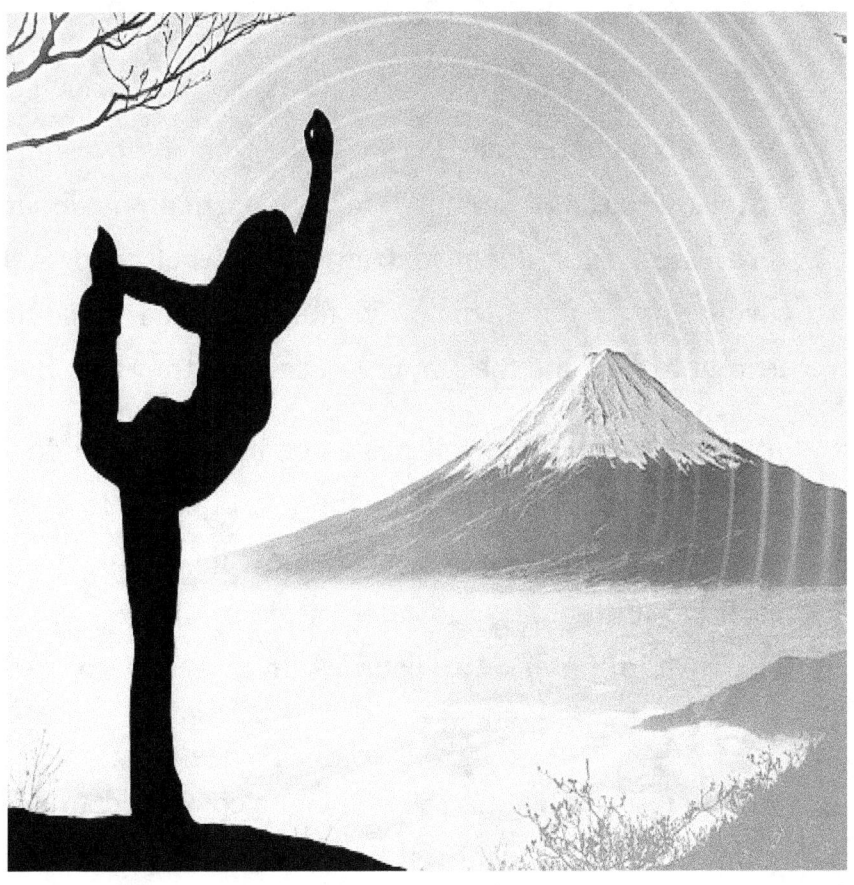

Achieving and sustaining the necessary body weight should be the aim of any eating pattern or food preferences. A person's body weight has been shown to be dependent on many environmental, genetic or even behavioral. One should maintain a focus on the balance of calories he intakes and as well, he or she expends. The calorie balance of a person is the relation between the calories the person intakes and that which he expends.

Even though people do not have control over the calories that is expended in the normal metabolic processes, they do have control on what food and drink they enjoy. This way, they are able to some extent to regulate the amount of calories they take in.

When the amount of calories taken in by an individual and that expended is zero, then there would be no gain or loss in weight by the individual whereas a positive difference indicates a gain in weight. A negative difference in calories indicates a loss of weight in the individual.

Maintaining a healthy body weight compared to the gain of body weight is actually more preferable. Therefore, one should aim at burning up more of the calories one intakes than one should expect to gain. People who are good at watching their weight shall be found to be equally good at the careful balance they take into account when consuming calories contained in the food they consume.

The current state of overweightness in the developed nations indicates ignorance on the side of the consumer on what to consume and in what amounts to consume what is available. The table below indicates the prevalence of obesity in the United States through the period of 2010. This is a problem since individuals with obesity problems have an increased chance of contracting other forms of diseases more readily than those without.

Unfortunately, these diseases- like cardiovascular diseases- are not specific to adults. Cardiovascular diseases can be seen in children and its signs is manifest even in adolescents with excess body fat.

Therefore, the primary target for a nation with a healthy eating timetable consists of targeting the young population first and foremost before anything else. This creates a welcome foundation not only for the future, but for the present as well since eating patterns among those of the younger generation can be guaranteed to spread as quickly as could have possibly been imagined before.

Maintaining a healthy diet is also relative to the subgroup of the population. For example,

- For women, it is necessary that they maintain a healthy and balanced weight before they become pregnant. This is necessary so that they avoid the risks of complications during the period of pregnancy.

- Pregnant women are encouraged to gain weight however, to a limit that is determined by professionals. Gaining weight beyond the acceptable limits may pose a health risk to the pregnant woman

- Those adults who fall in the age bracket of 65 years or older are restricted from activities leading to the gain of weight since weight loss at this stage is beneficial for the person

The environmental factors influencing the weight gain of an individual in the developed nations can be credited with the nature of obesity common in these countries. For example, in the modern working environment, there is increased outlets of foods that make it convenient for the buyer to enjoy a wide range of products from the menu. These products normally on offer are not severely checked by the consumer to determine the levels of nutrition they pose to benefit the individual but instead the individual judges their content by the sweetness they have often been found to have. Such environments promote the over consumption of calories and limited physical activity.

It is important to note that over the past decades, the average consumption; rather, the average number of calories available in the average American diet increased by approximately 600 calories. There have been increased portion sizes, with research showing that what is served at the present moment has a very high content of calories.

Communities with a larger number of fast food restaurants have been found to have a higher rate of BMI, compared with those with less. It has been documented that the number of fast food chains in the current century has doubled compared to the 1970s.

this has proven to create a nuisance in the food choices of Americans. For example, it has been found that a high number of people tend to eat out compared to the previous generations. Young adults and children tend to eat away from home, a culture slowly ingrained in the older generation by the fault of their sedentary natures and behaviors. Most Americans tend to be involved in little physical exercise compared to those in the previous decades majorly out of the changes in the workplaces and the shift in cultures, including the eating culture.

Since a majority of the population consumes food rich in calories that is higher than the recommended intake, there is a large increase in cases of being overweight being reported in the country. Among men and women older than 19, the average intake of calories tends to be 2640 and 1785 respectively. This number may not seem to be excessive or dangerous at all, but it is worth noting that many respondents in researches such as this tend to give incorrect answers for the sake of; sometimes, their privacy and their self esteem.

Calorie Balance: Food and Beverage Intake

It is important that one knows the amount of calories one intakes just so one can regulate the kinds of foods and beverages one consumes. This sort of calculation helps one to build an eating pattern while at the same time checking the weight and the level of calorie intake and expenditure. The biggest threat to accomplishing this; however, is that many Americans do not know what amount of calories they should or they are expected to consume in a day depending on the influencing factors.

Understanding Calorie Needs

The total number of calories an individual needs varies depending on a variety of factors including the height of the individual, the weight of the individual and even the age and the level of physical activities the individual partakes. The table below expounds on this, giving a clear picture of the exact measure of calories depending on the measure of a person's metrics.

TABLE 2-3. Estimated Calorie Needs per Day by Age, Gender, and Physical Activity Level[a]

Estimated amounts of calories needed to maintain calorie balance for various gender and age groups at three different levels of physical activity. The estimates are rounded to the nearest 200 calories. An individual's calorie needs may be higher or lower than these average estimates.

Gender	Age (years)	Physical Activity Level[b]		
		Sedentary	Moderately Active	Active
Child (female and male)	2-3	1,000-1,200[c]	1,000-1,400[c]	1,000-1,400[c]
Female[d]	4-8	1,200-1,400	1,400-1,600	1,400-1,800
	9-13	1,400-1,600	1,600-2,000	1,800-2,200
	14-18	1,800	2,000	2,400
	19-30	1,800-2,000	2,000-2,200	2,400
	31-50	1,800	2,000	2,200
	51+	1,600	1,800	2,000-2,200
Male	4-8	1,200-1,400	1,400-1,600	1,600-2,000
	9-13	1,600-2,000	1,800-2,200	2,000-2,600
	14-18	2,000-2,400	2,400-2,800	2,800-3,200
	19-30	2,400-2,600	2,600-2,800	3,000
	31-50	2,200-2,400	2,400-2,600	2,800-3,000
	51+	2,000-2,200	2,200-2,400	2,400-2,800

a. Data are drawn from analyses of usual dietary intakes conducted by the National Cancer Institute. Foods and beverages consumed were divided into 97 categories and ranked according to calorie contribution to the diet. Table shows each food category and its mean calorie contribution for each age group. Additional information on calorie contribution by age, gender, and race/ethnicity is available at

http://riskfactor.cancer.gov/diet/foodsources/.

b. Includes cake, cookies, pie, cobbler, sweet rolls, pastries, and donuts.

c. Includes white bread or rolls, mixed-grain bread, flavored bread, whole-wheat bread, and bagels.

d. Includes fried or baked chicken parts and chicken strips/patties, chicken stir-fries, chicken casseroles, chicken sandwiches, chicken salads, stewed chicken, and other chicken mixed dishes.

e. Sodas, energy drinks, sports drinks, and sweetened bottled water including vitamin water.

f. Includes macaroni and cheese, spaghetti, other pasta with or without sauces, filled pasta (e.g., lasagna and ravioli), and noodles.

g. Also includes nachos, quesadillas, and other Mexican mixed dishes.

h. Includes steak, meatloaf, beef with noodles, and beef stew.

i. Includes ice cream, frozen yogurt, sherbet, milk shakes, and pudding.

j. Includes peanut butter, peanuts, and mixed nuts.

k. Includes scrambled eggs, omelets, fried eggs, egg breakfast sandwiches/ biscuits, boiled and poached eggs, egg salad, deviled eggs, quiche, and egg substitutes.

l. Includes white rice, Spanish rice, and fried rice.

m. Includes fruit-flavored drinks, fruit juice drinks, and fruit punch.

n. Includes muffins, biscuits, and cornbread.

o. Fish other than tuna or shrimp.

Source: National Cancer Institute. Food sources of energy among U.S. population, 2005-2006. Risk Factor Monitoring and Methods. Control and Population Sciences. National Cancer Institute; 2010. http://riskfactor. cancer.gov/diet/foodsources/. Updated May 21, 2010. Accessed May 21, 2010.

Knowing one's calorie needs is necessary so one can compare the average intake one takes and that he or she ought to be taking. The best way to monitor this is therefore to check on one's body weight while adjusting the levels of intake depending on the change in the weight of the individual. Tracking one's body weight should not be a complicated task and adjusting that to the required amounts of calorie intake and expenditure should provide an easy way for one to monitor his or her calorie intake.

It is not to be taken with the ultimate strict measure that one must maintain a balance in the calorie intake. Maintaining a reasonable deficit is equally necessary for everybody. It does not matter, and it should not be of concern how this deficit is generated, for it might be out of the increased intake in calories or even out of increased rate of physical activity.

Carbohydrate, Protein, Fat and Alcohol

The above mentioned categories are the most common form of nutrients available in most diets. Most foods contain these in different combinations. Carbohydrates are the common source of calories in the diet of most people in the North American region. They can be either simple or complex. Simple carbohydrates include sugars whereas those in the complex category include starch and fibers. Some sugars are contained as natural compounds in foods whereas other forms of sugar are added to the food to make them seem like they contain sugars. An example is table sugar that is added to coffee and fructose corn syrup that is added to sugar sweetened beverages. Most carbohydrates; however, is consumed in terms of starches- common in foods such as potatoes, grains and starchy vegetables.

Starch may also be added to a variety of foods to refine or to stabilize them. Added sugars and starches generally provide calories but little of nutrients. Although people tend to consume an adequate amount of carbohydrates, they tend to consume these in the form of too much sugar and refined grain and very little in terms of fibers.

Proteins provide 4 calories per gram, just like carbohydrates. Proteins are found in wide range of animal and plant food. However, inadequate intake of proteins is quite rare in the northern parts of America.

Fats provide more calories per gram than the rest of the food groups. There are various types of fats including saturated, unsaturated, monounsaturated and trans fats. It is not common to find citizens of the United States with a deficiency of fats. However, most Americans consume trans fats compared to their consumption of unsaturated fats.

Alcohol; on the other hand, contains 7 calories per gram of it. Alcohol contains more calories and very little nutrients.

Macronutrient Proportion and Body Weight

To maintain their body weights, Americans have to ensure that their consumption of calories is within the range of AMDR. Studies have indicated that there is no optimal proportion of macronutrients that can facilitate the loss of weight or that can maintain the level of weight gain and weight loss.

Even though there has been recorded studies indicating that the level of intake of macronutrients ultimately leads to weight loss, this is only true as long as the individual makes effort to check on his rate of calorie intake. The total number of calories consumed is the essential dietary factor relevant to body weight. In adults, moderate evidence suggests that diets that are less than 45 percent of total calories as carbohydrate or more than 35 percent of total calories as protein are generally no more effective than other calorie-controlled diets for long-term weight loss and weight maintenance. Therefore, individuals who wish to lose weight or maintain weight loss can select eating patterns that maintain appropriate calorie intake and have macronutrient proportions that are within the AMDR ranges recommended in the Dietary Reference Intakes.

Individual Foods and Beverages and Body Weight

For the individual and in relation to the food that one consumes, one should aim at increasing the nutrients in foods one eats and focus on reducing the amount of foods that contain a high amount of calories. The following should be able to provide a guideline to individuals on how to limit the total number of calories they consume:

a) Increase intake of whole grains, vegetable and fruits in the daily meal routines. Studies have consistently indicated that adults who consume more whole grain foods appear to have a better grip at controlling their weight as compared to those adults who have less of whole grains in their diets.

b) Reduce the consumption of beverages sweetened with sugar. This helps in controlling the weight of the individuals. If not necessarily to avoid sweetened beverages, individuals should aim towards lowering the consumption of these beverages. Sugar added beverages are filled with high calorie substances and yet do not offer the individual enough of the nutrients the individual requires.

c) Monitor the intake of juice among children and young adults. Fruit juices are these days nothing but extracts coupled with added sugars, which as has been discussed, make it very difficult for individuals to acquire the nutrients they require while at the same time making it very easy for the same individuals to gain calories and in the long run to increase in weight.

d) Monitor the intake of alcoholic beverages among adults. As has been mentioned, there is a high rate of calorie intake among those who engage in the activities of drinking alcohol and hence this should be checked and put at a minimum considering the risks of gaining calories and being overweight that is obviously imminent

Studies have come to deny the existence of a relation between weight gain and products such as milk and poultry, beans and peas including soy with the total body weight of the individual.

Placing Individual Choice into an Overall Eating Pattern

It is difficult to restrict people to a strict meal pattern since eating habits tend to change with the coming of new generations. What people consume and what times they consume it is most often times tied to the culture they find themselves in. for example, it might be hard to dissociate snacks with movie goers, or more specifically- movie theaters. What this means is that new ways to handle the eating patterns of people must be adopted so as to create a guiding framework that will ultimately resonate with them.

One aspect of these that has been researched and substantial results documented is the measure of calories by the use of a standard referred to as calorie density- the unit of measurement representing the amount of calories for every unit measure of food. A dietary pattern low in calorie density is usually that involving a high number of fruits and vegetables in the diet and also that with high amounts of water and fiber. On the other hand, those foods with higher calorie densities include fatty foods.

Studies have suggested that foods low in calorie density improve weight management while those with higher calorie densities tend to increase the gain in weight among individuals. Although a limited or rather, a balanced intake of calories is good for the overall weight of an individual, it is necessary to consider as well the nutritional values of food. As has been mentioned with respect to carbohydrates, individuals should consider increasing their intake of naturally occurring carbohydrates such as whole grains, beans and peas.

Americans should move toward more healthful eating patterns. Overall, as long as foods and beverages consumed meet nutrient needs and calorie intake is appropriate, individuals can select an eating pattern that they enjoy and can maintain over time. Individuals should consider the calories from *all* foods and beverages they consume, regardless of when and where they eat or drink.

Physical activity is the other side of the calorie balance equation and should be considered when addressing weight management. In 2008, the U.S. Department of Health and Human Services released a comprehensive set of physical activity recommendations for Americans ages 6 years and older. Weight management along with health outcomes, including premature (early) death, diseases (such as coronary heart disease, type 2 diabetes, and osteoporosis), and risk factors for disease (such as high blood pressure and high blood cholesterol) were among the outcomes considered in developing the *2008 Physical Activity Guidelines for Americans*. Getting adequate amounts of physical activity conveys many health benefits independent of body weight.

Strong evidence supports that regular participation in physical activity also helps people maintain a healthy weight and prevent excess weight gain. Further, physical activity, particularly when combined with reduced calorie intake, may aid weight loss and maintenance of weight loss. Decreasing time spent in sedentary behaviors also is important as well. Strong evidence shows that more screen time, particularly television viewing, is associated with overweight and obesity in children, adolescents, and adults. Substituting active pursuits for sedentary time can help people manage their weight and provides other health benefits.

The *2008 Physical Activity Guidelines for Americans* provides guidance to help Americans improve their health, including weight management, through appropriate physical activity (see Table 2-5). The amount of physical activity necessary to successfully maintain a healthy body weight depends on calorie intake and varies considerably among adults, including older adults. To achieve and maintain a healthy body weight, adults should do the equivalent[40] of 150 minutes of moderate-intensity aerobic activity each week. If necessary, adults should increase their weekly minutes of aerobic physical activity gradually over time and decrease calorie intake to a point where they can achieve calorie balance and a healthy weight. Some adults will need a higher level of physical activity than others to achieve and maintain a healthy body weight. Some may need more than the equivalent of 300 minutes per week of moderate-intensity activity.

For children and adolescents ages 6 years and older, 60 minutes or more of physical activity per day is recommended. Although the Physical Activity Guidelines do not include a specific quantitative recommendation for children ages 2 to 5 years, young children should play actively several times each day. Children and adolescents are often active in short bursts of time rather than for sustained periods of time, and these short bursts can add up to meet physical activity needs. Physical activities for children and adolescents of all ages should be developmentally appropriate and enjoyable, and should offer variety.

Principles for Controlling Calorie Balance and Weight

The best method of regulating the calorie balance and the weight of individuals with regard to the foods consumed is to check on the levels of ignorance and thereby to increase the awareness of individuals with regard to the food they consume. The table below shows the physical activity guidelines that can be adopted by individuals to increase their level of awareness on their weight and put it in check with regard to a healthy or simply to healthy physical exercises.

age group	guidelines
Below 17 years	Children and adolescents should do 60 minutes (1 hour) or more of physical

	activity daily. • Aerobic: Most of the 60 or more minutes a day should be either moderatea- or vigorousb- intensity aerobic physical activity, and should include vigorous- intensity physical activity at least 3 days a week. • Muscle- strengthening: c As part of their 60 or more minutes

	of daily physical activity, children and adolescents should include muscle-strengthening physical activity on at least 3 days of the week. • Bone-strengthening: d As part of their 60 or more minutes of daily physical activity, children and adolescents should include bone-

	strengthening physical activity on at least 3 days of the week. • It is important to encourage young people to participate in physical activities that are appropriate for their age, that are enjoyable, and that offer variety.
17-35 years	• All adults should avoid inactivity. Some physical activity is

	better than none, and adults who participate in any amount of physical activity gain some health benefits.
	• For substantial health benefits, adults should do at least 150 minutes (2 hours and 30 minutes) a week of moderate-intensity, or 75 minutes (1 hour and 15 minutes) a week of

| | vigorous-intensity aerobic physical activity, or an equivalent combination of moderate- and vigorous-intensity aerobic activity. Aerobic activity should be performed in episodes of at least 10 minutes, and preferably, it should be spread throughout the week.

• For |
| --- | --- |

	additional and more extensive health benefits, adults should increase their aerobic physical activity to 300 minutes (5 hours) a week of moderate-intensity, or 150 minutes a week of vigorous-intensity aerobic physical activity, or an equivalent combination of moderate- and vigorous-intensity activity.

	Additional health benefits are gained by engaging in physical activity beyond this amount. • Adults should also include muscle-strengthening activities that involve all major muscle groups on 2 or more days a week.
Above 35 years	• Older adults should follow the adult guidelines. When older adults cannot

	meet the adult guide-lines, they should be as physically active as their abilities and conditions will allow.
	• Older adults should do exercises that maintain or improve balance if they are at risk of falling.
	• Older adults should determine their level of effort for physical activity relative to their level of

	fitness.
	• Older adults with chronic conditions should understand whether and how their conditions affect their ability to do regular physical activity safely.
a. Moderate-intensity physical activity: Aerobic activity that increases a person's heart rate and breathing to some extent. On a scale relative to a person's capacity, moderate-intensity activity is usually a 5 or 6 on a 0 to 10 scale. Brisk walking, dancing, swimming, or bicycling on a level terrain are	

examples.

b. Vigorous-intensity physical activity: Aerobic activity that greatly increases a person's heart rate and breathing. On a scale relative to a person's capacity, vigorous-intensity activity is usually a 7 or 8 on a 0 to 10 scale. Jogging, singles tennis, swimming continuous laps, or bicycling uphill are examples.

c. Muscle-strengthening activity: Physical activity, including exercise that increases skeletal muscle strength, power, endurance, and mass. It includes strength training, resistance training, and muscular strength and endurance exercises.

d. Bone-strengthening activity: Physical activity that produces an impact or tension force on bones, which promotes bone growth and strength. Running, jumping rope,

and lifting weights are examples. Source: Adapted from U.S. Department of Health and Human Services. 2008 Physical Activity Guidelines for Americans. Washington (DC): U.S. Department of Health and Human Services; 2008. ODPHP Publication No. U0036. http://www.health.gov/paguideline s. Accessed August 12, 2010.	

Chapter 3: Foods and Food Components to Cut Down

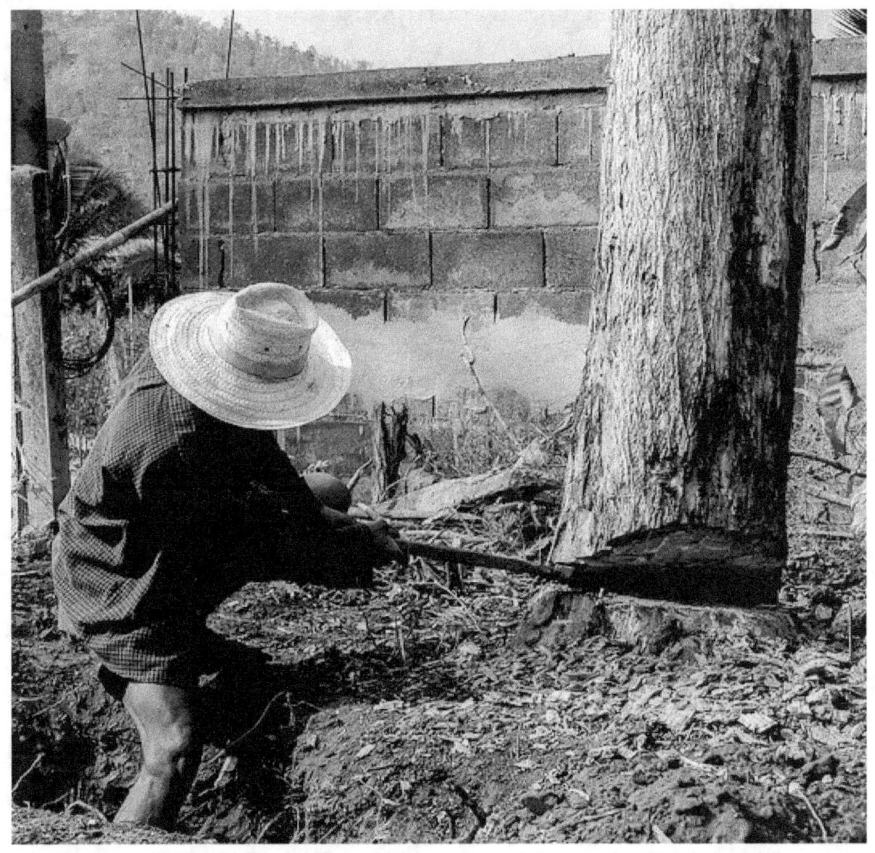

Currently, very few Americans consume diets that meet Dietary Guideline recommendations. This chapter focuses on certain foods and food components that are consumed in excessive amounts and may increase the risk of certain chronic diseases. These include sodium, solid fats (major sources of saturated and *trans* fatty acids), added sugars, and refined grains. These food components are consumed in excess by children, adolescents, adults, and older adults. In addition, the diets of most men exceed the recommendation for cholesterol. Some people also consume too much alcohol.

This excessive intake replaces nutrient-dense forms of foods in the diet, making it difficult for people to achieve recommended nutrient intake and control calorie intake. Many Americans are overweight or obese, and are at higher risk of chronic diseases, such as cardiovascular disease, diabetes, and certain types of cancer. Even in the absence of overweight or obesity, consuming too much sodium, solid fats, saturated and *trans* fatty acids, cholesterol, added sugars, and alcohol increases the risk of some of the most common chronic diseases in the United States. Discussing solid fats in addition to saturated and *trans* fatty acids is important because, apart from the effects of saturated and *trans* fatty acids on cardiovascular disease risk, solid fats are abundant in the diets of Americans and contribute significantly to excess calorie intake. The recommendations in this chapter are based on evidence that eating less of these foods and food components can help Americans meet their nutritional needs within appropriate calorie levels, as well as help reduce chronic disease risk.

Recommendations

Reduce daily sodium intake to less than 2,300 milligrams (mg) and further reduce intake to 1,500 mg among persons who are 51 and older and those of any age who are African American or have hypertension, diabetes, or chronic kidney disease. The 1,500 mg recommendation applies to about half of the U.S. population, including children, and the majority of adults.

Consume less than 10 percent of calories from saturated fatty acids by replacing them with monounsaturated and polyunsaturated fatty acids.

Consume less than 300 mg per day of dietary cholesterol.

Keep *trans* fatty acid consumption as low as possible, especially by limiting foods that contain synthetic sources of *trans* fats, such as partially hydrogenated oils, and by limiting other solid fats.

Reduce the intake of calories from solid fats and added sugars.

Limit the consumption of foods that contain refined grains, especially refined grain foods that contain solid fats, added sugars, and sodium.

If alcohol is consumed, it should be consumed in moderation—up to one drink per day for women and two drinks per day for men—and only by adults of legal drinking age.

Sodium

Sodium is an essential nutrient and is needed by the body in relatively small quantities, provided that substantial sweating does not occur. On average, the higher an individual's sodium intake, the higher the individual's blood pressure. A strong body of evidence in adults documents that as sodium intake decreases, so does blood pressure. Moderate evidence in children also has documented that as sodium intake decreases, so does blood pressure. Keeping blood pressure in the normal range reduces an individual's risk of cardiovascular disease, congestive heart failure, and kidney disease. Therefore, adults and children should limit their intake of sodium.

Fats

Dietary fats are found in both plant and animal foods. Fats supply calories and essential fatty acids, and help in the absorption of the fat-soluble vitamins A, D, E, and K. The IOM established acceptable ranges for total fat intake for children and adults (children ages 1 to 3 years: 30–40% of calories; children and adolescents ages 4 to 18 years: 25–35%; adults ages 19 years and older: 20–35%).

Fatty acids are categorized as being saturated, monounsaturated, or polyunsaturated. Fats contain a mixture of these different kinds of fatty acids. *Trans* fatty acids are unsaturated fatty acids. However, they are structurally different from the predominant unsaturated fatty acids that occur naturally in plant foods and have dissimilar health effects.

The types of fatty acids consumed are more important in influencing the risk of cardiovascular disease than is the total amount of fat in the diet. Animal fats tend to have a higher proportion of saturated fatty acids (seafood being the major exception), and plant foods tend to have a higher proportion of monounsaturated and/or polyunsaturated fatty acids (coconut oil, palm kernel oil, and palm oil being the exceptions)

Most fats with a high percentage of saturated or *trans* fatty acids are solid at room temperature and are referred to as "solid fats," while those with more unsaturated fatty acids are usually liquid at room temperature and are referred to as "oils." Solid fats are found in most animal foods but also can be made from vegetable oils through the process of hydrogenation, as described below.

Saturated Fatty Acids

The body uses some saturated fatty acids for physiological and structural functions, but it makes more than enough to meet those needs. People therefore have no dietary requirement for saturated fatty acids. A strong body of evidence indicates that higher intake of most dietary saturated fatty acids is associated with higher levels of blood total cholesterol and low-density lipoprotein (LDL) cholesterol. Higher total and LDL cholesterol levels are risk factors for cardiovascular disease.

Consuming less than 10 percent of calories from saturated fatty acids and replacing them with monounsaturated and/or polyunsaturated fatty acids is associated with low blood cholesterol levels, and therefore a lower risk of cardiovascular disease. Lowering the percentage of calories from dietary saturated fatty acids even more, to 7 percent of calories, can further reduce the risk of cardiovascular

Despite longstanding recommendations on total fat, saturated fatty acids, and cholesterol, intakes of these fats have changed little from 1990 through 2005–2006, the latest time period for which estimates are available. Total fat intake contributes an average of 34 percent of calories. The following sections provide details on types of fat to limit in the diet.

FIGURE 3-3. Fatty Acid Profiles of Common Fats and Oils

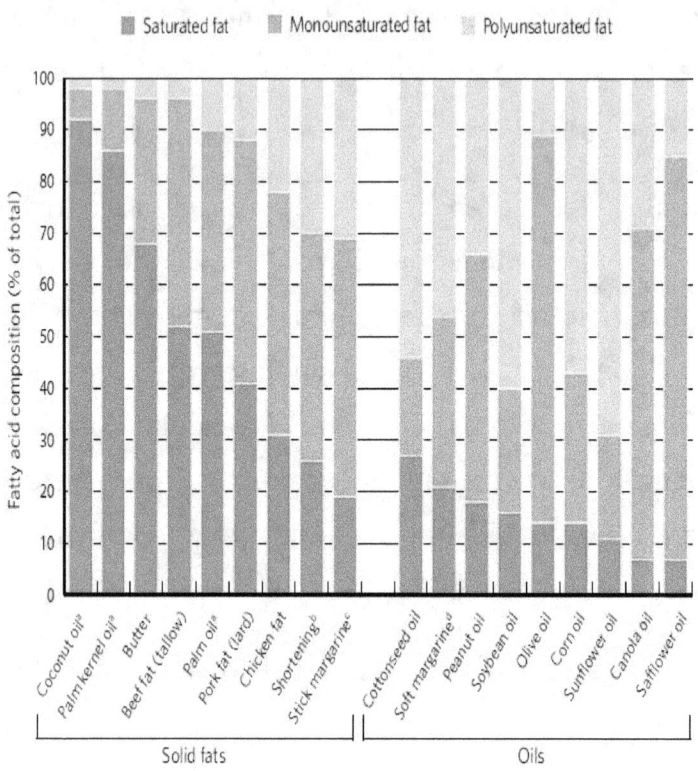

a. Coconut oil, palm kernel oil, and palm oil are called oils because they come from plants. However, they are semi-solid at room temperature due to their high content of short-chain saturated fatty acids. They are considered solid fats for nutritional purposes.

b. Partially hydrogenated vegetable oil shortening, which contains *trans* fats.

c. Most stick margarines contain partially hydrogenated vegetable oil, a source of *trans* fats.

d. The primary ingredient in soft margarine with no *trans* fats is liquid vegetable oil.

Source: U.S. Department of Agriculture, Agricultural Research Service, Nutrient Data Laboratory. USDA National Nutrient Database for Standard Reference, Release 22, 2009. Available at http://www.ars.usda.gov/ba/ bhnrc/ndl. Accessed July 19, 2010.

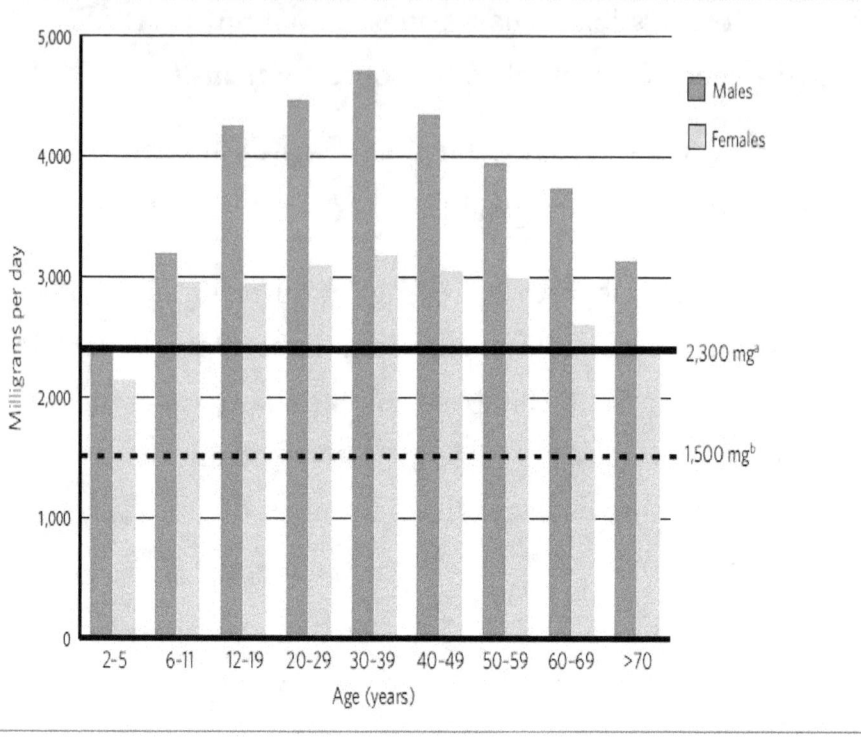

FIGURE 3-1. Estimated Mean Daily Sodium Intake, by Age-Gender Group, NHANES 2005-2006

a. 2,300 mg/day is the Tolerable Upper Intake Level (UL) for sodium intake in adults set by the Institute of Medicine (IOM). For children younger than age 14 years, the UL is less than 2,300 mg/day.

b. 1,500 mg/day is the Adequate Intake (AI) for individuals ages 9 years and older.

Source: U.S. Department of Agriculture, Agricultural Research Service and U.S. Department of Health and Human Services, Centers for Disease Control and Prevention. What We Eat In America, NHANES 2005–2006.
http://www.ars.usda.gov/Services/docs.htm?docid= 13793. Accessed August 11, 2010.

Consuming less than 10 percent of calories from saturated fatty acids and replacing them with monounsaturated and/or polyunsaturated fatty acids is associated with low blood cholesterol levels, and therefore a lower risk of cardiovascular disease. Lowering the percentage of calories from dietary saturated fatty acids even more, to 7 percent of calories, can further reduce the risk of cardiovascular disease. Saturated fatty acids contribute an average of 11 percent of calories to the diet, which is higher than recommended. Major sources of saturated fatty acids in the American diet include regular (full-fat) cheese (9% of total saturated fat intake); pizza (6%); grain-based desserts[48] (6%); dairy-based desserts[49] (6%);

chicken and chicken mixed dishes (6%); and sausage, franks, bacon, and ribs (5%).

Transfatty acids

Trans fatty acids are found naturally in some foods and are formed during food processing; they are not essential in the diet. A number of studies have observed an association between increased *trans* fatty acid intake and increased risk of cardiovascular disease. This increased risk is due, in part, to its LDL cholesterol-raising effect. Therefore, Americans should keep their intake of *trans* fatty acids as low as possible.

Some *trans* fatty acids that Americans consume are produced by a process referred to as hydrogenation. Hydrogenation is used by food manufacturers to make products containing unsaturated fatty acids solid at room temperature (i.e., more saturated) and therefore more resistant to becoming spoiled or rancid. Partial hydrogenation means that some, but not all, unsaturated fatty acids are converted to saturated fatty acids; some of the unsaturated fatty acids are changed from a *cis* to *trans* configuration. *Trans* fatty acids produced this way are referred to as "synthetic" or "industrial" *trans* fatty acids. Synthetic *trans* fatty acids are found in the partially hydrogenated oils used in some margarines, snack foods, and prepared desserts as a replacement for saturated fatty acids. *Trans* fatty acids also are produced by grazing animals, and small quantities are therefore found in meat and milk products.[50] These are called "natural" or "ruminant" *trans* fatty acids. There is limited evidence to conclude whether synthetic and natural *trans* fatty acids differ in their metabolic effects and health outcomes. Overall, synthetic *trans* fatty acid levels in the U.S. food supply have decreased dramatically since 2006 when the declaration of the amount of *trans* fatty acids on the Nutrition Facts label became mandatory. Consuming fat-free or low-fat milk and milk products and lean meats and poultry will reduce the intake of natural *trans* fatty acids. Because natural *trans* fatty acids are present in meat, milk, and milk products,[50] their elimination is not recommended because this could have potential implications for nutrient adequacy.

Added Sugars

Sugars are found naturally in fruits (fructose) and fluid milk and milk products (lactose). The majority of sugars in typical American diets are sugars added to foods during processing, preparation, or at the table. These "added sugars" sweeten the flavor of foods and beverages and improve their palatability. They also are added to foods for preservation purposes and to provide functional attributes, such as viscosity, texture, body, and browning capacity.

Although the body's response to sugars does not depend on whether they are naturally present in food or added to foods, sugars found naturally in foods are part of the food's total package of nutrients and other healthful components. In contrast, many foods that contain added sugars often supply calories, but few or no essential nutrients and no dietary fiber. Both naturally occurring sugars and added sugars increase the risk of dental caries.

As a percent of calories from total added sugars, the major sources of added sugars in the diets of Americans are soda, energy drinks, and sports drinks (36% of added sugar intake), grain-based desserts

(13%), sugar-sweetened fruit drinks[54] (10%), dairy-based desserts (6%), and candy (6%) (Figure 3-6).

Reducing the consumption of these sources of added sugars will lower the calorie content of the diet, without compromising its nutrient adequacy. Sweetened foods and beverages can be replaced with those that have no or are low in added sugars. For example, sweetened beverages can be replaced with water and unsweetened beverages.

Why Calories from fats and added sugars are a particular concern

Solid fats and added sugars are consumed in excessive amounts, and their intake should be limited. Together, they contribute a substantial portion of the calories consumed by Americans—35 percent on average, or nearly 800 calories per day—without contributing importantly to overall nutrient adequacy of the diet. Moreover, they have implications for weight management. Foods containing solid fats and added sugars are no more likely to contribute to weight gain than any other source of calories in an eating pattern that is within calorie limits. However, as the amount of solid fats and/or added sugars increases in the diet, it becomes more difficult to also eat foods with sufficient dietary fiber and essential vitamins and minerals, and still stay within calorie limits. For most people, no more than about 5 to 15 percent of calories from solid fats and added sugars can be reasonably accommodated in the USDA Food Patterns, which are designed to meet nutrient needs within calorie limits.

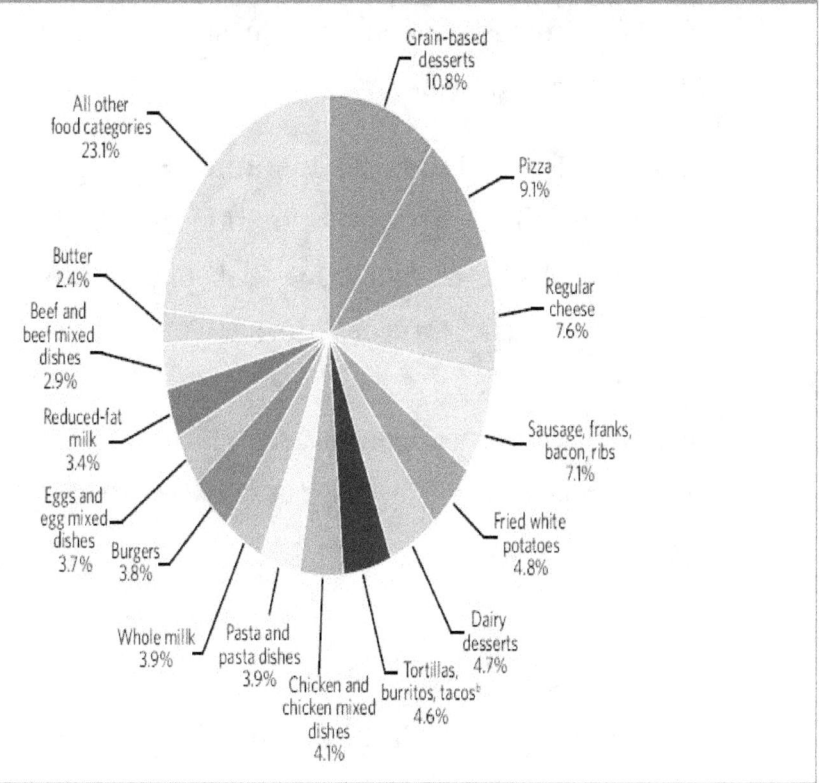

FIGURE 3-5. Sources of Solid Fats in the Diets of the U.S. Population Ages 2 Years and Older, NHANES 2003-2004[a]

Grain-based desserts 10.8%

Pizza 9.1%

Regular cheese 7.6%

Sausage, franks, bacon, ribs 7.1%

Fried white potatoes 4.8%

Dairy desserts 4.7%

Tortillas, burritos, tacos[b] 4.6%

Chicken and chicken mixed dishes 4.1%

Pasta and pasta dishes 3.9%

Whole milk 3.9%

Burgers 3.8%

Eggs and egg mixed dishes 3.7%

Reduced-fat milk 3.4%

Beef and beef mixed dishes 2.9%

Butter 2.4%

All other food categories 23.1%

a. Data are drawn from analyses of usual dietary intake conducted by the National Cancer Institute. Foods and beverages consumed were divided into 97 categories and ranked according to solid fat contribution to the diet. "All other food categories" represents food categories that each contributes less than 2% of the total solid fat intake.

b. Also includes nachos, quesadillas, and other Mexican mixed dishes.

Source: National Cancer Institute. Sources of solid fats in the diets of U.S. population ages 2 years and older, NHANES 2003-2004. Risk Factor Monitoring and Methods. Cancer Control and Population Sciences. http://riskfactor.cancer.gov/diet/foodsources/food_groups/table3.html. Accessed August 11, 2010.

Refined Grains

The refining of whole grains involves a process that results in the loss of vitamins, minerals, and dietary fiber. Most refined grains are enriched with iron, thiamin, riboflavin, niacin, and folic acid before being further used as ingredients in foods. This returns some, but not all, of the vitamins and minerals that were removed during the refining process. Dietary fiber and some vitamins and minerals that are present in whole grains are not routinely added back to refined grains. Unlike solid fats and added sugars, enriched refined grain products have a positive role in providing some vitamins and minerals. However, when consumed beyond recommended levels, they commonly provide excess calories, especially because many refined grain products also are high in solid fats and added sugars (e.g., cookies and cakes).

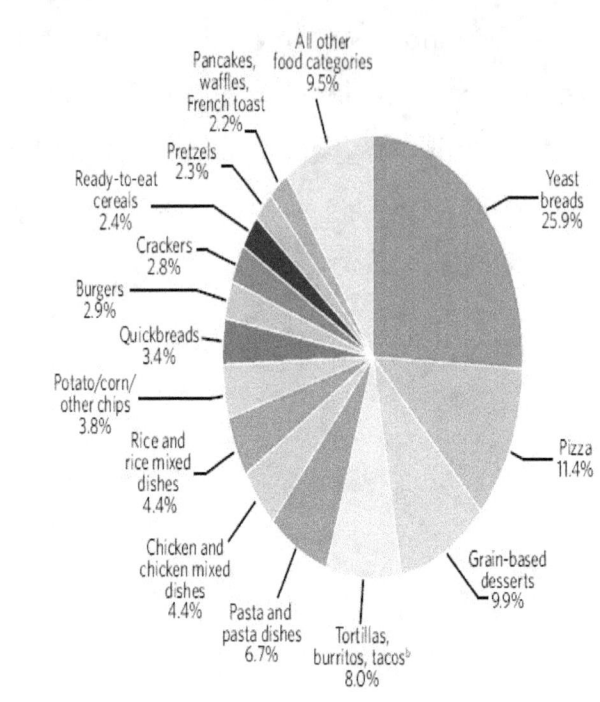

a. Data are drawn from analyses of usual dietary intake conducted by the National Cancer Institute. Foods and beverages consumed were divided into 97 categories and ranked according to refined grain contribution to the diet. "All other food categories" represents food categories that each contributes less *than 2% of the total intake of refined grains. b. Also includes nachos, quesadillas, and other Mexican mixed dishes.*

Source: National Cancer Institute. Sources of refined grains in the diets of the U.S. population ages 2 years and older, NHANES 2003–2004. Risk Factor Monitoring and Methods. Cancer Control and Population Sciences. http://riskfactor.cancer.gov/diet/foodsources/food_ groups/table3.html. Accessed August 11, 2010.

Alcohol

In the United States, approximately 50 percent of adults are current regular drinkers and 14 percent are current infrequent drinkers. An estimated 9 percent of men consume an average of more than two drinks per day and 4 percent of women consume an average of more than one drink per day. Of those who drink, about 29 percent of U.S. adult drinkers report binge drinking within the past month, usually on multiple occasions. This results in about 1.5 billion episodes of binge drinking in the United States each year.

The consumption of alcohol can have beneficial or harmful effects, depending on the amount consumed, age, and other characteristics of the person consuming the alcohol. Alcohol consumption may have beneficial effects when consumed in moderation. Strong evidence from observational studies has shown that moderate alcohol consumption is associated with a lower risk of cardiovascular disease. Moderate alcohol consumption also is associated with reduced risk of all-cause mortality among middle-aged and older adults and may help to keep cognitive function intact with age. However, it is not recommended that anyone begin drinking or drink more frequently on the basis of potential health benefits because moderate alcohol intake also is associated with increased risk of breast cancer, violence, drowning, and injuries from falls and motor vehicle crashes.

Because of the substantial evidence clearly demonstrating the health benefits of breastfeeding, occasionally consuming an alcoholic drink does not warrant stopping breastfeeding. However, breastfeeding women should be very cautious about drinking alcohol, if they choose to drink at all. If the infant's breastfeeding behavior is well established, consistent, and predictable (no earlier than at 3 months of age), a mother may consume a single alcoholic drink if she then waits at least 4 hours before breastfeeding. Alternatively, she may express breast milk before consuming the drink and feed the expressed milk to her infant later.

key definitions for alcohol

What is moderate alcohol consumption? Moderate alcohol consumption is defined as up to 1 drink per day for women and up to 2 drinks per day for men.

What is heavy or high-risk drinking? Heavy or high-risk drinking is the consumption of more than 3 drinks on any day or more than 7 per week for women and more than 4 drinks on any day or more than 14 per week for men.

What is binge drinking? Binge drinking is the consumption within 2 hours of 4 or more drinks for women and 5 or more drinks for men.

Excessive (i.e., heavy, high-risk, or binge) drinking has no benefits, and the hazards of heavy alcohol intake are well known. Excessive drinking increases the risk of cirrhosis of the liver, hypertension, stroke, type 2 diabetes, cancer of the upper gastrointesti-nal tract and colon, injury, and violence. Excessive drinking over time is associated with increased body weight and can impair short-and long-term cognitive function. For the growing percentage of the population with elevated blood pressure, reducing alcohol intake can effectively lower blood pres-sure, although this is most effective when paired with changes in diet and physical activity patterns. Excessive alcohol consumption is responsible for an average of 79,000 deaths in the United States each year. More than half of these deaths are due to binge drinking. Binge drinking also is associated with a wide range of other health and social problems, including sexually transmitted diseases, unintended pregnancy, and violent crime.

Try to eat less salt – no more than 6g a day for adults

Get active and try to be a healthy weight

Drink plenty of water

Don't skip breakfast

Bread, rice, potatoes, pasta and other starchy foods

Fruit and vegetables

Milk and dairy foods

Meat, fish, eggs, beans and other non-dairy sources of protein

Foods and drinks in the fifth group, i.e. those high in fat and/or sugar, can be consumed sparingly as part of a healthy balanced diet but should not be eaten instead of foods/drinks from the other food groups, or too often or in large amounts. Having a variety of foods in the diet is important for health – it is not necessary to follow the model at every meal, but rather over a day or two.

Beans and Peas

Beans and peas are the mature forms of legumes. They include kidney beans, pinto beans, black beans, garbanzo beans (chickpeas), lima beans, black-eyed peas, split peas, and lentils.

Beans and peas are excellent sources of protein. They also provide other nutrients, such as iron and zinc, similar to seafood, meat, and poultry. They are excellent sources of dietary fiber and nutrients such as potassium and folate, which also are found in other vegetables.

Because of their high nutrient content, beans and peas may be considered both as a vegetable and as a protein food. Individuals can count beans and peas as either a vegetable or a protein food.

Green peas and green (string) beans are not considered to be "Beans and Peas." Green peas are similar to other starchy vegetables and are grouped with them. Green beans are grouped with other vegetables such as onions, lettuce, celery, and cabbage because their nutrient content is similar to those foods.

What is the difference between the various types of grains?

Whole grains include the entire grain seed, usually called the kernel. The kernel consists of three components—the bran, germ, and endosperm. If the kernel has been cracked, crushed, or flaked, then, to be called a "whole grain" a food must retain the same relative proportions of these components as they exist in the intact grain. Whole grains are consumed either as a single food (e.g., wild rice or popcorn) or as an ingredient in foods (e.g., in cereals, breads, and crackers). Some examples of whole-grain ingredients include buckwheat, bulgur, millet, oatmeal, quinoa, rolled oats, brown or wild rice, whole-grain barley, whole rye, and whole wheat.

Refined grains have been milled to remove the bran and germ from the grain. This is done to give grains a finer texture and improve their shelf life, but it also removes dietary fiber, iron, and many B vitamins.

Enriched grains are grain products with B vitamins (thiamin, riboflavin, niacin, folic acid) and iron added. Most refined-grain products are enriched.

Milk and milk products contribute many nutrients, such as calcium, vitamin D (for products fortified with vita-min D), and potassium, to the diet. Moderate evidence shows that intake of milk and milk products is linked to improved bone health, especially in children and adolescents. Moderate evidence also indicates that intake of milk and milk products is associated with a reduced risk of cardiovascular disease and type 2 diabetes and with lower blood pressure in adults.

Protein foods include seafood, meat, poultry, eggs, beans and peas, soy products, nuts, and seeds. In addition to protein, these foods contribute B vitamins (e.g., niacin, thiamin, riboflavin, and B6), vitamin E, iron, zinc, and magnesium to the diet. However, protein also is found in some foods that are classified in other food groups (e.g., milk and milk products). The fats in meat, poultry, and eggs are considered solid fats, while the fats in seafood, nuts, and seeds are considered oils. Meat and poultry should be con-sumed in lean forms to decrease intake of solid fats.

Nutrients of Concern

Dietary fiber is the non-digestible form of carbohydrates and lignin. Dietary fiber naturally occurs in plants, helps provide a feeling of fullness, and is important in promoting healthy laxation. Some of the best sources of dietary fiber are beans and peas, such as navy beans, split peas, lentils, pinto beans, and black beans. Additional sources of dietary fiber include other vegetables, fruits, whole grains, and nuts. All of these foods are consumed below recommended levels in the typical American diet. Bran, although not a whole grain, is an excellent source of dietary fiber.

Adequate calcium status is important for optimal bone health. In addition, calcium serves vital roles in nerve transmission, constriction and dilation of blood vessels, and muscle contraction. A significant number of Americans have low bone mass, a risk factor for osteoporosis, which places them at risk of bone fractures. Age groups of particular concern due to low calcium intake from food include children ages 9 years and older, adolescent girls, adult women, as well as adults ages 51 years and older. All ages are encouraged to meet their Recommended Dietary Allowance (RDA) for calcium.

Building Healthy Eating Patterns

Individuals and families can incorporate the recommendations presented in each of the previous chapters into an overall healthy way to eat—a healthy eating pattern.71 A growing body of evidence from research on eating patterns supports these recommendations. A healthy eating pattern is not a rigid prescription, but rather an array of options that can accommodate cultural, ethnic, traditional, and personal preferences and food cost and avail-ability. Americans have flexibility in making choices to create a healthy eating pattern that meets nutrient needs and stays within calorie limits.

Conclusion

In conclusion therefore, the awareness with regard to the foods consumed among population the world over must be brought to the front. This should be done since the food industry is quickly revolutionizing the way people consume food and not only that, the way people make choices on what food to take and what not.

The current food industries in the developing nations have overturned the general view with regard to food and this should be restricted based on the values adopted in the family setting. Since most patterns relating to the intake of foods and most societies adopt various ways of food preferences with regard to culture, there should and must be a policy that restricts the careless intake of substandard food (that is, food not beneficial in terms of nutrients) and to add to such strict policy, the players in the market working in the diverse food industry must as well account to the relevant government organs mandated to oversee the industry. The reason this must be done is so as to restrict players who in the long run disrupt the habits of not only the society as a whole but as individuals taken singly.

Appendix

The table indicates the type of food in the first column, the Key consumer behavior in the second column and the potential strategies to counter these behaviors in the third column.

WHOLE GRAINS	Increase whole-grain intake. Consume at least half of all grains as whole grains.	Eat a variety of foods from the protein foods group each week. This group includes seafood, beans and peas, and nuts, as well as lean meats, poultry, and eggs. Eat seafood in place of meat or poultry twice a week. Select some seafood that is higher in oils and lower in mercury, such as salmon, trout, and herring. Select lean meats and poultry. Choose meat cuts that are low in fat and ground beef that is extra

		lean (at least 90% lean). Trim or drain fat from meat and remove poultry skin before cooking or eating. Try grilling, broiling, poaching, or roasting. These cooking methods do not add extra fat. Drain fat from ground meats after cooking. Avoid breading on meat and poultry, which adds calories.
REFINED GRAINS	Whenever possible, replace refined grains with whole grains.	Eat fewer refined grain products, especially those that are high in calories from solid fats and/or added sugars, such as cakes, cookies, other desserts, and pizza. Replace white bread, rolls, bagels, muffins, pasta, and rice with whole-grain versions.

		When choosing a refined grain, check the ingredients list to make sure it is made with enriched flour.
OILS	Use oils instead of solid fats, when possible.	When using spreads, choose soft margarines with zero *trans* fats made from liquid vegetable oil, rather than stick margarine or butter. If you do use butter, use only a small amount. When cooking, use vegetable oils such as olive, canola, corn, safflower, or sunflower oil rather than solid fats (butter, stick margarine, shortening, lard). Consider calories when adding oils to foods or in cooking. Use only small amounts to keep calories in check. Use the

		ingredients list to choose foods that contain oils with more unsaturated fats. Use the Nutrition Facts label to choose foods that contain less saturated fat.
SOLID FATS	Cut back on solid fats. Choose foods with little solid fats and prepare foods to minimize the amount of solid fats. Limit saturated fat intake	Eat fewer foods that contain solid fats. The major sources for Americans are cakes, cookies, and other desserts (often made with butter, margarine, or shortening); pizza; cheese; processed and fatty meats (e.g., sausages, hot dogs, bacon, ribs); and ice cream. Select lean meats and poultry, and fat-free or low-fat milk and milk products. When cooking, replace solid fats such as butter, beef fat,

	and keep *trans* fat intake as low as possible.	chicken fat, lard, stick margarine, and shortening with oils; or choose cooking methods that do not add fat. Choose baked, steamed, or broiled rather than fried foods most often. Check the Nutrition Facts label to choose foods with little or no saturated fat and no *trans* fat. Limit foods containing partially hydrogenated oils, a major source of *trans* fats.
ADDED SUGAR	Cut back on foods and drinks with added sugars or caloric sweeteners (sugar-	Drink few or no regular sodas, sports drinks, energy drinks, and fruit drinks. Eat less cake, cookies, ice cream, other desserts, and candy. If you do have these foods and drinks, have a small portion. These drinks

| | sweetened beverages) . | and foods are the major sources of added sugars for Americans. Choose water, fat-free milk, 100% fruit juice, or unsweetened tea or coffee as drinks rather than sugar-sweetened drinks. Select fruit for dessert. Eat less of high-calorie desserts. Use the Nutrition Facts label to choose breakfast cereals and other packaged foods with less total sugars, and use the ingredients list to choose foods with little or no added sugars. |
| SODIUM | Reduce sodium intake. Choose foods low | Use the Nutrition Facts label to choose foods lower in sodium. When purchasing canned foods, select those labeled as |

	in sodium and prepare foods with little salt. Increase potassium intake.	"reduced sodium," "low sodium," or "no salt added." Rinse regular canned foods to remove some sodium. Many packaged foods contain more sodium than their made-from-fresh counterparts. Use little or no salt when cooking or eating. Trade in your salt shaker for the pepper shaker. Spices, herbs, and lemon juice can be used as alternatives to salt to season foods with a variety of flavors. Gradually reduce the amount of sodium in your foods. Your taste for salt will change over time. Get more potassium in your diet. Food sources of potassium include potatoes, cantaloupe, bananas,

		beans, and yogurt.
ALCOHOL	For adults of legal drinking age who choose to drink alcohol, consume it in moderation. Avoid alcohol in certain situations that can put you at risk.	Limit alcohol to no more than 1 drink per day for women and 2 drinks per day for men. Avoid excessive (heavy or binge) drinking. Consider the calorie content of mixers as well as the alcohol. If breastfeeding, wait at least 4 hours after drinking alcohol before breastfeeding. Alcohol should not be consumed at all until consistent latch on and breastfeeding patterns are established. Avoid alcohol if you are pregnant or may become pregnant; if under the legal drinking age; if you are on medication that can

		interact with alcohol; if you have medical conditions that could be worsened by drinking; and if planning to drive, operate machinery, or do other activities that could put you at risk if you are impaired. Do not begin drinking or drink more frequently on the basis of potential health benefits.
FOOD SAFETY	Be food safe.	Clean: Wash hands, utensils, and cutting boards before and after contact with raw meat, poultry, seafood, and eggs. Separate: Keep raw meat and poultry apart from foods that won't be cooked. Cook: Use a food thermometer. You can't tell if food is cooked safely by

TYPE OF FOOD	KEY CONSUMER BEHAVIORS	POTENTIAL STRATEGIES
		how it looks. Chill: Chill leftovers and takeout foods within 2 hours and keep the refrigerator at 40°F or below.
CALORIE INTAKE	Consume foods and drinks to meet, not exceed, calorie needs.	Know your calorie needs. See Table 2-3 and Appendix 6 for estimates. Weigh yourself and adjust what and how much you eat and/or your physical activity based on your weight change over time.

	Track food and calorie intake.	Track what you eat using a food journal or an online food planner (e.g., http://www.mypyramidtra cker.gov). Check the calories and servings per package on the Nutrition Facts label. For foods and drinks that do not have a label or posted calorie counts, try an online calorie counter. Pay attention to feelings of hunger. Eat only until you are satisfied, not full. If you tend to overeat, be aware of time of day, place, and your mood while eating so you can better control the amount you eat. Limit eating while watching television, which can result in overeating. If you choose to eat while watching television, portion out a

		small serving.
	Cook and eat more meals at home, instead of eating out.	Cook and eat at home more often, preferably as a family. When preparing meals, include vegetables, fruits, whole grains, fat-free or low-fat dairy products, and protein foods that provide fewer calories and more nutrients. Experiment with healthy recipes and ingredient substitutions.
PHYSICAL ACTIVITY	Increase physical activity.	Pick activities you like and that fit into your life. For children, activity should be fun and developmentally appropriate. Be active with family and friends. Having a support network can help you stay active. Keep track of your physical activity and gradually increase it to

		meet the recommendations of the *2008 Physical Activity Guidelines for Americans.* Physical activity can be tracked at http://www.presidentschall enge.org or by using logs like the one found at http://www.health.gov/pag uidelines.
	Slowly build up the amount of physical activity you choose.	Start by being active for longer each time; then do more by being active more often.
VEGETAB LES	Increase vegetable	Include vegetables in meals and in snacks. Fresh,

intake. Eat recommended amounts of vegetables, and include a variety of vegetables, especially dark-green vegetables, red and orange vegetables, and beans and peas.	frozen, and canned vegetables all count. When eating canned vegetables, choose those labeled as reduced sodium or no salt-added. Add dark-green, red, and orange vegetables to soups, stews, casseroles, stir-fries, and other main and side dishes. Use dark leafy greens, such as romaine lettuce and spinach, to make salads. Focus on dietary fiber—beans and peas are a great source. Add beans or peas to salads (e.g., kidney or garbanzo beans), soups (e.g., split peas or lentils), and side dishes (e.g., baked beans or pinto beans), or serve as a main dish. Keep raw, cut-up vegetables handy for quick snacks. If

| | | serving with a dip, choose lower calorie options, such as yogurt-based dressings or hummus, instead of sour cream or cream cheese-based dips. When eating out, choose a vegetable as a side dish. With cooked vegetables, request that they be prepared with little or no fat and salt. With salads, ask for the dressing on the side so you can decide how much you use. When adding sauces, condiments, or dressings to vegetables, use small amounts and look for lower calorie options (e.g., reduced-fat cheese sauce or fat-free dressing). Sauces can make vegetables more appealing, but often add extra calories. |

PROTEIN FOODS	Choose a variety of foods from the protein foods group. Increase the amount and variety of seafood consumed by choosing seafood in place of some meat and poultry.	Eat a variety of foods from the protein foods group each week. This group includes seafood, beans and peas, and nuts, as well as lean meats, poultry, and eggs. Eat seafood in place of meat or poultry twice a week. Select some seafood that is higher in oils and lower in mercury, such as salmon, trout, and herring. Select lean meats and poultry. Choose meat cuts that are low in fat and ground beef that is extra lean (at least 90% lean). Trim or drain fat from meat and remove poultry skin before cooking or eating. Try grilling, broiling, poaching, or roasting. These cooking methods do

		not add extra fat. Drain fat from ground meats after cooking. Avoid breading on meat and poultry, which adds calories.

www.ingramcontent.com/pod-product-compliance
Lightning Source LLC
Chambersburg PA
CBHW071211280526
45787CB00002B/641